Tumescent Liposuction

Gerald H. Pitman, M.D., F.A.C.S.

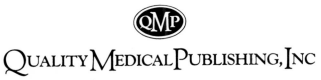

QUALITY MEDICAL PUBLISHING, INC

St. Louis, Missouri
1995

Every effort has been made to ensure the accuracy of the drug information provided in this book; however, the health care professional is legally responsible for verifying the dosage requirements with the manufacturers' package inserts and is thus advised. The author uses dosages of drugs at variance with recommendations in the drug manufacturers' package inserts. The author has found such usage safe and effective in his own practice. The health care professional is cautioned, however, that lidocaine and epinephrine can be toxic drugs and that administration of large volumes of fluid can cause circulatory and respiratory decompensation. The individual practitioner must determine safety and efficacy under the conditions of his own practice.

Printed in the United States of America

Quality Medical Publishing, Inc.
11970 Borman Dr., Suite 222
St. Louis, Missouri 63146

ISBN   0-942219-95-3

QM/IPC/IPC
5   4   3   2   1

The tumescent technique is the infiltration of copious amounts of dilute lidocaine and epinephrine into the subcutaneous fat prior to liposuction. Enough fluid is injected so that the tissues become swollen and firm (hence the name "tumescent"). Although the technique was initially developed to permit liposuction under local anesthesia,[1] its benefits extend beyond pain ablation.

The four major advantages of the tumescent technique are decreased blood loss and bruising, replenishment of fluid, enhanced local anesthesia, and enlargement of the subcutaneous space.

Reduced Blood Loss and Bruising. Blood loss can be reduced to negligible amounts for most patients. In a personal series of 116 operations with a mean aspirate volume of 1877 ml (range 1000 to 4150 ml), mean estimated blood loss (EBL) was less than 14% of the aspirate.[2] Stated another way, for every 1000 ml of aspirate, the average patient lost 140 ml of whole blood. EBL was calculated from pre- and postoperative hematocrit levels and estimated blood volume. The method of calculation has been previously described.[3]

Most of the 116 operations were performed with the patient under sedation or general anesthesia, but a subset of 22 procedures were done using pure local anesthesia (no sedatives or narcotics). The mean aspirate volume for operations under pure local anesthesia was 1705 ml (1000 to 4150 ml). The average blood loss was less than 2% of aspirate for the 22 operations performed under pure local anesthesia.

I believe that the incremental decrease in blood loss under pure local anesthesia occurred in the following way. In order to achieve total tissue anesthesia without narcotics or sedation, the local solution was completely dispersed through the subcutaneous fat. Total saturation of the tissues with the lidocaine-epinephrine solution produced not just a profound tissue anesthesia but also a more intense vasoconstriction. Hence the decreased blood loss.

For most patients, the differences in blood loss between complete and near-complete saturation of the tissues with the lidocaine-epinephrine solution are unimportant. For patients undergoing very high volume liposuction (>5000 ml), a meticulous and complete saturation of the fat with the epinephrine-containing solution becomes more important. I avoid operating on patients requiring more than 5000 ml aspirations because I believe they frequently obtain inferior cosmetic results and are usually better served by exercise and weight loss regimens.

Although I did not perform a controlled double-blind study, it is my strong clinical impression that postoperative bruising and swelling are also significantly reduced in patients treated with tumescent liposuction.

[1]Klein JA. Tumescent technique for local anesthesia improves safety in large-volume liposuction. Plast Reconstr Surg 92:1085-1098, 1993.

[2]Pitman GH. Tumescent liposuction, a surgeon's perspective (in preparation).

[3]Pitman GH, Holzer J. Safe suction. Fluid replacement and blood loss parameters. Perspect Plast Surg 5(1):79-89, 1991.

Reduction of Intravenous Fluid Requirements. Intravenous fluid requirements are reduced or eliminated as the large volume of injectate is absorbed into the circulation by hypodermoclysis. My patients receive an average volume of subcutaneous injection equal to twice the total aspirate. This 2:1 ratio of injectate to aspirate provides complete fluid replacement. In fact, provision of large volumes of additional intravenous fluid can result in dangerous fluid overload.

During tumescent liposuction, the anesthesiologist limits intravenous fluids to the minimum amount necessary to maintain venous access and provide medication. This volume is commonly less than 100 ml and never more than 500 ml. At the conclusion of the operation, I calculate the sum of: (1) fluids injected into the subcutaneous space plus (2) fluids delivered via the intravenous route. If total fluid administration has been less than twice the volume of aspirate, the patient is given enough intravenous fluids in the immediate postoperative period so that total perioperative delivery of fluids (subcutaneous plus intravenous) is twice the volume of aspirate. If the sum of intraoperative subcutaneous plus intravenous fluids is equal to or greater than twice the volume of aspirate, no additional fluids are given.

Enhanced Local Anesthesia. Large volumes of dilute lidocaine can provide profound anesthesia in the entire operative area during surgery and well into the postoperative period. Anesthesia persists for as long as 12 hours. The need for postoperative narcotics is significantly reduced or eliminated. Patients are frequently able to leave the recovery area and return home without pain medication.

Patients having general anesthesia or sedation also benefit from the preoperative infiltration of lidocaine-containing solutions since systemic analgesic requirements are reduced in the intraoperative and postoperative periods.

Enlargement of the Subcutaneous Space. Distention of the tissues by the large volume of injectate results in a hydrodissection that amplifies the volume of the subcutaneous space, permitting suction closer to the surface of the skin, facilitating more precise removal of small fat collections, and minimizing skin surface irregularities.

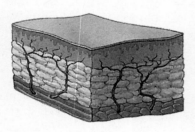
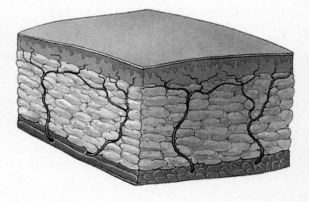

Volume enlargement of the fat compartment is analogous to visual enlargement of the operative field when using loupe or microscopic magnification. The distention produced by hydrodissection also enlarges the space between fibrous elements, eases passage of the cannula, decreases tissue trauma, and reduces the surgeon's effort.

TECHNIQUE

Copious volumes of dilute lidocaine with epinephrine are infiltrated into the subcutaneous space using hypodermic needles and infiltrating cannulas. There is no fixed volume required for each anatomic area. Rather, infiltration is complete when the tissues are uniformly distended and firm and the skin is pallid from vasoconstriction.

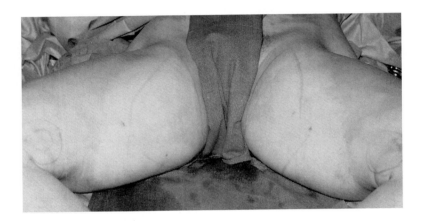

Although there is no absolute formula for injection, I have found that a solution of 0.05% lidocaine with 1:1,000,000 epinephrine provides profound tissue anesthesia and intense vasoconstriction. The solution is conveniently made by adding the necessary ingredients to a 1000 ml bag of lactated Ringer's solution for injection.

2% lidocaine	25.0 ml
8.4% (1 mEq/ml) sodium bicarbonate	2.5 ml
1:1000 epinephrine	1.0 ml
Lactated Ringer's solution	1000.0 ml
0.05% lidocaine with 1:1,000,000 epinephrine	1029.0 ml

The manufacturer acidifies lidocaine prior to shipping to prolong shelf life. Since injection of an acid solution creates stinging, I add sodium bicarbonate to neutralize the acidity. Sodium bicarbonate, 8.4%, added to commercial lidocaine in a volumetric ratio of 1:10 produces a neutral solution.[4] The solution should be made up immediately before use and should not be stored.

[4]McKay W, Morris R, Mushlin P. Sodium bicarbonate attenuates pain on skin infiltration with lidocaine with or without epinephrine. Anesth Analg 66:572-574, 1987.

Warming the injectate to body temperature prior to infiltration maintains patient comfort and prevents hypothermia. A microwave oven is convenient for heating the injectate.

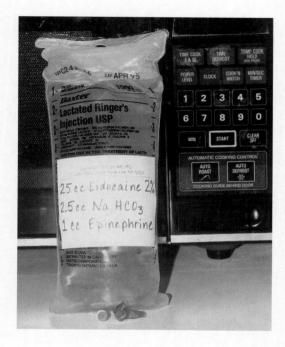

If the patient is awake, induction of complete anesthesia begins with injection of a local solution using a 30-gauge hypodermic needle on a 10 ml syringe. Skin wheals are raised at multiple access sites surrounding the area to be treated.

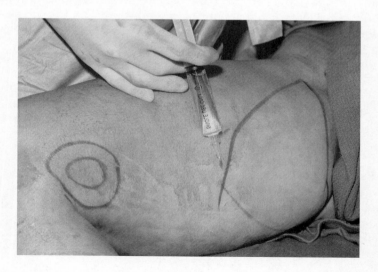

After access sites are numb, additional injections are given via a 20-gauge 3.5-inch spinal needle attached to sterile intravenous tubing brought into the operative field from an intravenous bag filled with the solution for injection.

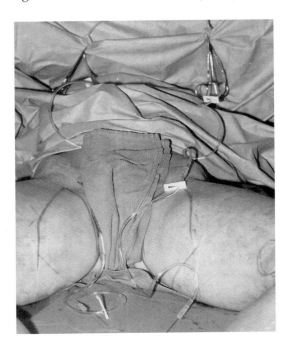

Pressurized infusors powered by nitrogen or carbon dioxide permit convenient and rapid infiltration. Each infusor holds two 1000 ml bags.

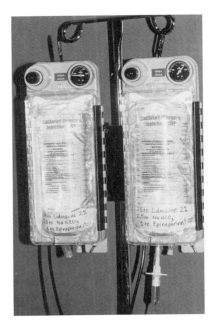

Hand-pumped pressure infusors such as those used for rapid blood infusion provide a less convenient yet less expensive alternative. The hand-pumped infusors are shown in the videotape.

Spinal needles passed through the anesthetized access sites deliver the initial fluids to the operative area to provide a partial level of anesthesia.

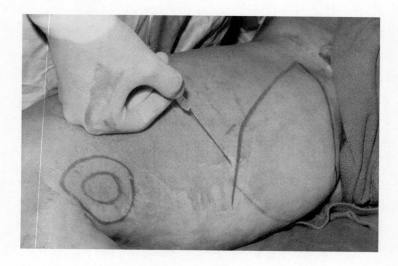

Once partial anesthesia is achieved, infiltrating cannulas are passed through stab wounds. Large volumes of anesthetic solution may be deposited rapidly into the fat. The cannulas have a Luer-Lok fitting at the proximal end and have multiple perforations at the distal end. The cannulas are 25 cm long and either 2 or 3 mm in outside diameter.

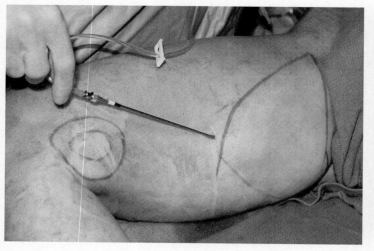
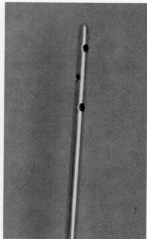

The initial cannula injection is made in the deep fat. More superficial tissues should be infiltrated last. The patient below is shown before and after infiltration with local anesthesia. Note the swelling and pallor of the tissues, which are firm to the touch.

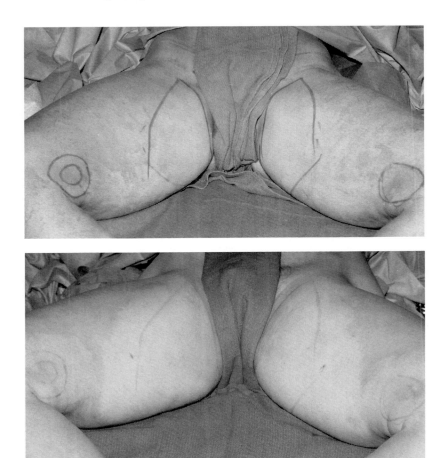

Infiltration volumes in each area vary, depending on the size of the patient, the size of the area, and the amount of fat in the area. Typical volumes are shown below.

INFILTRATION VOLUMES

Submental	100-200 ml
Abdomen	500-2000 ml
Hip/flank, each side	300-800 ml
Lateral thigh, each side	500-1000 ml
Medial thigh, each side	250-500 ml
Knee, each side	100-200 ml
Calf and ankle, each side	500-1000 ml

In the awake patient it is important to test for complete anesthesia by passing the largest size cannula to be used into the fat before starting suction. If anesthesia is incomplete, more local solution needs to be added to the operative site. Testing and additional infiltration should be accomplished before starting suction. Once suction has started, the normal tissue architecture is destroyed, and it is more difficult to achieve local anesthesia.

If the surgeon wishes to perform the procedure on an awake patient, little or no sedatives should be given so that the patient can cooperate when being tested for complete anesthesia. In an awake patient the infiltrate should be injected slowly initially so as not to cause pain from rapid tissue distention. Once partial anesthesia has been achieved, additional infiltration can proceed more rapidly. Nevertheless, achievement of complete anesthesia in an awake patient can require 45 minutes or longer. If the patient is under general anesthesia or under deep sedation, infiltration can be performed more rapidly. For the patient under general anesthesia, the surgeon can dispense with a 20-gauge hypodermic needle and proceed directly to rapid infiltration with the cannula.

The tumescent technique expands the volume of the fat compartment and temporarily converts small fat compartments into larger ones. The net effect is that fine cannulas can be moved more easily in the expanded compartment. Moreover, instead of having to work directly adjacent to the dermal layer, the surgeon can place the fine cannulas at a slightly deeper level but still close to the skin surface. Expansion of the fat compartment reduces the likelihood of creating surface irregularities.

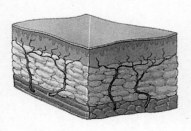 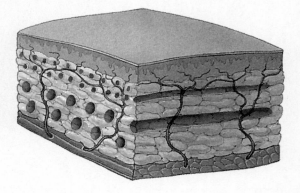

When the tumescent technique is used, the aspirate will consist largely of pure white fat. After setting in the collection bottle for 30 minutes, the fat separates into an upper fat fraction and a lower fluid fraction stained red by small amounts of blood.

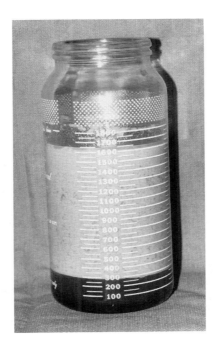

In my personal series of patients,[5] the average fat fraction has been approximately 80% of aspirate. The remaining 20% is water containing small amounts of blood. Areas suctioned shortly after infiltration yield aspirates containing larger volumes of water. Aspirates from areas suctioned later contain smaller volumes of water.

Since the tissues are distended by the tumescent technique, the surgeon must modify his evaluation of end point. There will be an increased volume of aspirate at the end of the procedure, and the pinch test will be slightly thicker than usual due to increased water in the tissues.

Since there is little bleeding and the fat flows easily through the cannula, there may be a tendency to overresect when first using this technique. The surgeon first learning tumescent liposuction is advised to be conservative and leave more tissue in situ than with other techniques.

[5]Pitman GH. Tumescent liposuction, a surgeon's perspective (in preparation).

This patient was treated with tumescent liposuction with a good result in all areas except the hips, which show evidence of overresection. She is shown before and 6 months after liposuction of the hips, thighs, and knees.

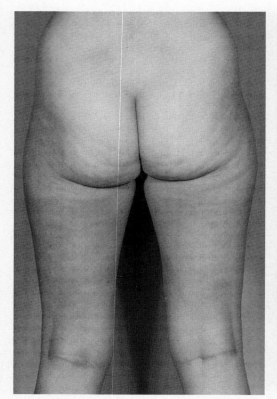
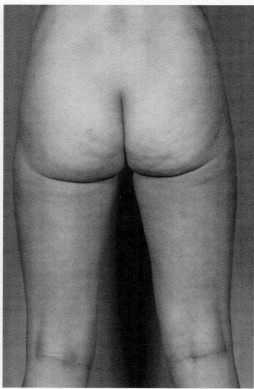

This 19-year-old woman is shown before and 3 days after liposuction of 2000 ml from her thighs, buttocks, and knees using the tumescent technique. There is almost no bruising in the postoperative view. Because swelling is also decreased with tumescent liposuction, some improvement in contour is already evident. The fullness at the top of the medial thighs is the result of swelling above the top of the compressive garment.

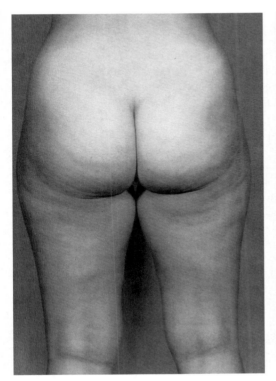 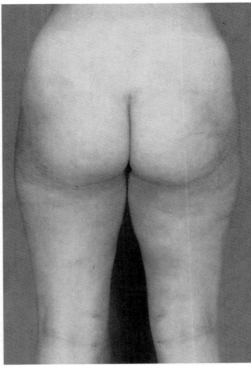

PHARMACOKINETICS

Patients undergoing tumescent liposuction receive doses of lidocaine far in excess of the manufacturer's recommended maximum dose of 7 mg/kg.[6] In 98 patients in whom I recorded the lidocaine dose, the mean was 31 mg/kg (10.0 to 48.6 mg/kg).[7] Despite these high doses of lidocaine, no patient had a serious toxic reaction. To understand why toxic reactions did not occur, one must consider the pharmacokinetics of lidocaine as used in the tumescent technique.

Lidocaine toxicity does not occur unless plasma lidocaine levels exceed the patient's toxic threshold. Subjective toxicity such as drowsiness, anxiety, or restlessness may occur at the upper levels of the therapeutic range (3 to 5 µg/ml). Tremors and other objective toxic signs do not occur until levels exceed 5 µg/ml. More serious and life-threatening toxicity can occur at levels exceeding 8 µg/ml.

PLASMA LIDOCAINE LEVELS AND TOXICITY

Therapeutic level	1-5 µg/ml
Subjective toxicity	3-6 µg/ml
Objective toxicity	5-9 µg/ml
Seizures, cardiac depression	8-12 µg/ml
Coma	12 µg/ml
Respiratory arrest	20 µg/ml
Cardiac arrest	26 µg/ml

When dilute lidocaine mixed with epinephrine is infiltrated into the subcutaneous tissues in the manner described above, lidocaine is avidly bound to the tissues and only slowly released into the circulation where it is metabolized by the liver and excreted by the kidneys. Toxic plasma levels are not reached. Moreover, because of slow release from the tissues, peak plasma lidocaine levels do not occur until approximately 12 hours following injection. Delayed release of lidocaine from tissues at the injection site also explains the prolonged duration of local anesthesia after surgery.

Since maintenance of plasma lidocaine levels below the toxic threshold is dependent on normal hepatic and renal function, use of the tumescent technique in patients with functional impairments of these organs should be critically evaluated. The technique should be modified or eliminated in these individuals.

[6]Physician's Desk Reference, 49th ed. Montvale, N.J.: Medical Economics, 1995, p 582.
[7]Pitman GH. Tumescent liposuction, a surgeon's perspective (in preparation).

In an interesting case study, Klein[8] injected the subcutaneous fat of a patient with dilute lidocaine with epinephrine at a dose of 35 mg/kg. He then measured serial serum lidocaine levels. No liposuction was performed (upper line in chart). The maximal serum lidocaine level was less than 2.5 µg/ml and occurred 14 hours after injection. Klein injected the same solution into the same patient 3 weeks later and then performed liposuction. The maximum serum lidocaine level was slightly less than 2 µg/ml and occurred 11 hours after injection.

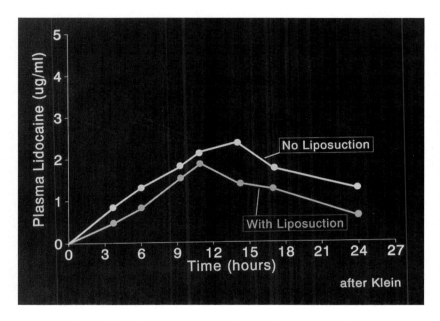

Modified from Klein JA. Tumescent technique for local anesthesia improves safety in large-volume liposuction. Plast Reconstr Surg 92:1085-1098, 1993.

This study demonstrated that if the tumescent technique is used properly, plasma lidocaine levels do not reach toxic thresholds, peak plasmal lidocaine levels occur approximately 12 hours after injection, and removal of lidocaine from the tissues by liposuction plays only a minor role in reducing plasma lidocaine levels. Other investigators have shown a similar time course and low levels of serum lidocaine when using the tumescent technique.[9]

---

[8]Klein JA. Tumescent technique for local anesthesia improves safety in large-volume liposuction. Plast Reconstr Surg 92:1085-1098, 1993.

[9]Samdal F, Amland P, Bugge J. Plasma lidocaine levels during suction-assisted lipectomy using large doses of dilute lidocaine with epinephrine. Plast Reconstr Surg 92:1217-1222, 1993.

I obtained serum lidocaine levels 12 hours after surgery in 16 patients who underwent liposuction.[10] Twelve-hour serum lidocaine levels were positively correlated with lidocaine dose, and a lidocaine dose of 40 mg/kg can be expected to produce a 12-hour serum lidocaine level of 2.6 µg/ml (+ 0.5 µg/ml).

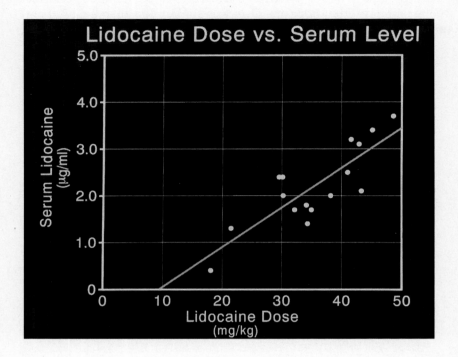

Since a lidocaine dose of 40 mg/kg will, in my hands, produce a 12-hour serum lidocaine level of approximately 2.6 µg/ml, I am comfortable using this dosage in all patients. Therefore I have constructed a 40 mg/kg isodose graph that I keep in the operating room for ready reference.

[10]Klein JA. Tumescent technique for local anesthesia improves safety in large-volume liposuction. Plast Reconstr Surg 92:1085-1098, 1993.

This graph correlates weight of the patient with volume of subcutaneous injection. For every patient weight there is a volume of subcutaneous injection that will give the patient a 40 mg/kg dose of lidocaine. For example, a patient weighing 50 kg will receive a lidocaine dose of 40 mg/kg if injected with 4000 ml. A 100 kg patient, on the other hand, will require an injection of 8000 ml to receive a lidocaine dose of 40 mg/kg. *Note that each 1000 ml of injectate contains 500 mg of lidocaine, 1 mg of epinephrine, and 2.5 mEq of sodium bicarbonate.*

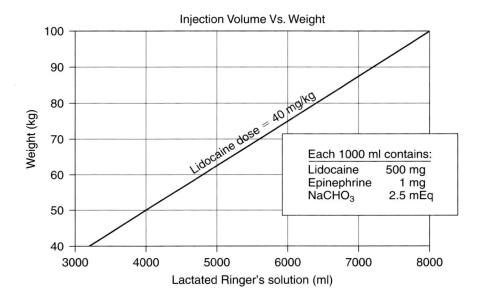

I have used as much as 50 mg/kg in some patients without untoward effect, but each surgeon must determine safe dose limits for his own patients when using this technique. These exceptionally large doses of lidocaine have been tolerated safely by large numbers of patients under the conditions described above, that is, injection into the subcutaneous fat of lidocaine and epinephrine in an ultradilute solution.

DISADVANTAGES

The tumescent technique does have some disadvantages. When a pure local is used as the sole form of anesthesia (no narcotics, sedative, or general anesthetic), tumescent liposuction requires a prolonged period for injection. It is, therefore, unsuitable as a pure modality for the anxious patient. Moreover, a patient who is calm at the beginning of the procedure may find prolonged and repeated injections unpleasant and, in fact, intolerable. Except for relatively small areas, I have found that it is best to have an anesthesiologist available in all instances. With an anesthesiologist in attendance, all patients have a pleasant, safe, and pain-free operation. Furthermore, the cosmetic result is never compromised because of a restless or uncomfortable patient. The tumescent technique may also be unsuitable if a thin patient is undergoing treatment of multiple areas since the dosage necessary for complete anesthesia may produce unacceptably high plasma lidocaine levels.

For all patients, whether under pure local, local with sedation, or general anesthesia, use of tumescent liposuction requires modification of the surgeon's technique. The tensely distended operative area has a different feel and consistency, and the pinch test at end point may be somewhat thicker than expected. Since the aspirate contains an increased amount of fluid due to the large volume of injectate, aspirate volumes will be higher with this technique. Also, since there is little or no blood in the aspirate and the extraction of tissue is more facile, there may be a tendency to remove too much fat. When first using this technique, the surgeon should perform resection conservatively until he has acquired greater experience.

CASE REPORTS

Tumescent liposuction is applicable to a broad range of patients, from those who require small, subtle resections to those needing very large resections.

This 30-year-old woman was 5 feet 7 inches tall and weighed 130 pounds. She desired reduction of her lateral and medial thighs. I used the tumescent technique with the patient under pure local anesthesia (no sedatives or narcotics).

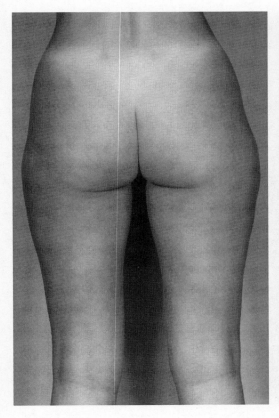 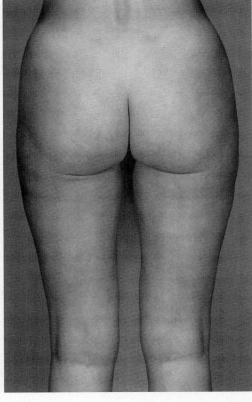

After giving a 4000 ml subcutaneous injection, I removed 100 ml from each medial thigh, 450 ml from the left lateral thigh, and 500 ml from the right lateral thigh. She is shown before and 8 months following treatment.

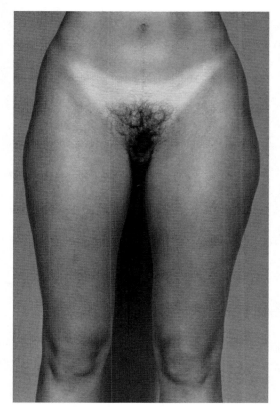
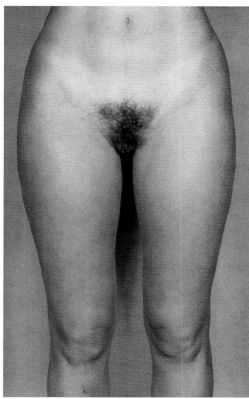

This 34-year-old woman was 5 feet 2 inches tall and weighed 123 pounds. Her waist and trochanteric circumferences were 24 inches and 41 inches, respectively. She considered herself 10 pounds over her ideal weight, but even at her lowest weight her thighs were disproportionately full. I performed liposuction using the tumescent technique with the patient under general anesthesia. I injected 4000 ml into the subcutaneous tissues. She is shown before and 6 months following removal of 150 ml from each medial thigh, 800 ml from the left lateral thigh, 600 ml from the right lateral thigh, and 50 ml from each knee.

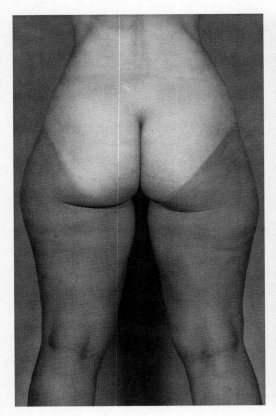 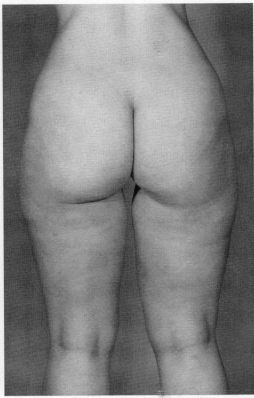

The postoperative trochanteric circumference was reduced to 38 inches. The patient requested additional liposuction, which I performed using the tumescent technique with the patient under general anesthesia. At her second operation I removed 500 ml from each lateral thigh, 125 ml from the left medial thigh, and 250 ml from the right medial thigh. The patient was pleased with the final result but did not return for additional photographs.

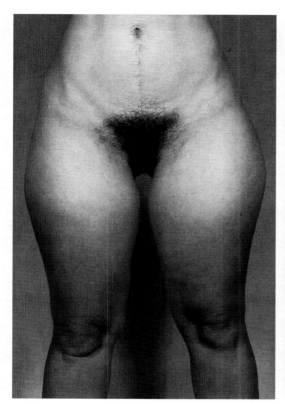 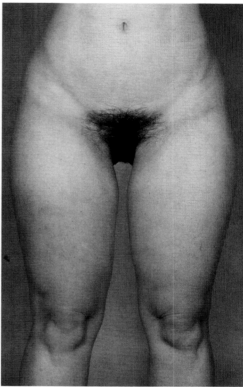

CONCLUSION

The tumescent technique enhances liposuction by reducing blood loss, bruising, and swelling. The need for blood transfusion has been eliminated in my practice even for patients undergoing 5000 ml aspirations. The tumescent technique also is a complete method of fluid replacement, obviating the need for intravenous volume support. For some patients, surgery is performed under pure local anesthesia with no sedatives or narcotics. For all patients, pain is reduced and recovery is accelerated. Finally, by enlarging the subcutaneous space, tumescence eases passage of the cannula, speeds aspiration, and facilitates smooth liposuction of the superficial layer.

Once mastered, tumescent liposuction is a valuable addition to the surgeon's technique. It permits outstanding aesthetic results with increased patient safety and comfort.